WƓ

Speaking Up for Myself

Sheila Hollins, Jackie Downer, Linette Farquarson and Oyepeju Raji
illustrated by Lisa Kopper

Books Beyond Words
RCPsych Pꞁ ꓳn
LONDON

First edition 2002, Gaskell/St George's Hospital Medical School.

Reprinted with amendments 2009, RCPsych Publications/St George's, University of London.

Text and illustrations © Sheila Hollins & Lisa Kopper 2002, 2009.

ISBN 978-1-901242-79-9

British Library Cataloguing-in-Publication Data

A catalogue record for this book is available from the British Library.

Distributed in North America by Publishers Storage and Shipping Company.

Printed and bound by ArtQuarters Press Limited, London.

The Royal College of Psychiatrists is a charity registered in England and Wales (228636) and in Scotland (SC038369). St George's Hospital Charity is a registered charity (no. 241527).

Further information about the Books Beyond Words series can be obtained from: Royal College of Psychiatrists, 17 Belgrave Square, London SW1X 8PG (tel: 020 7235 2351; fax 020 7245 1231; website www.rcpsych.ac.uk/bbw).

Authors

Sheila Hollins is Professor of Psychiatry of Learning Disability at St George's Hospital Medical School, University of London; Jackie Downer is a self-advocate and trainer at St George's Hospital Medical School; Linette Farquarson is an independent advocate who has supported people with learning/intellectual disabilities in a variety of settings; Oyepeju Raji is specialist registrar in psychiatry of learning disability at St George's.

Lisa Kopper is a distinguished illustrator of children's books and is well known for her clear style and ability to draw feelings as well as form.

Acknowledgements

We would like to thank our editorial advisors, Sandra Montague, Wendy Perez, Alice Richards, Richard West and members of Wandsworth Rathbone, for helping us to think of ideas for the book and for telling us what was needed in the pictures.

We were very grateful to Thelma Bennett for giving us valuable editorial feedback before her very sad death in 2001.

We would also like to thank Ellen Clifford from 'Speak Out Project' (Wandsworth Care Alliance) and Shahnaaz Docherty from Wandsworth Rathbone for their support and input to the project.

Finally, we are grateful to the Department of Health for their generous financial support.

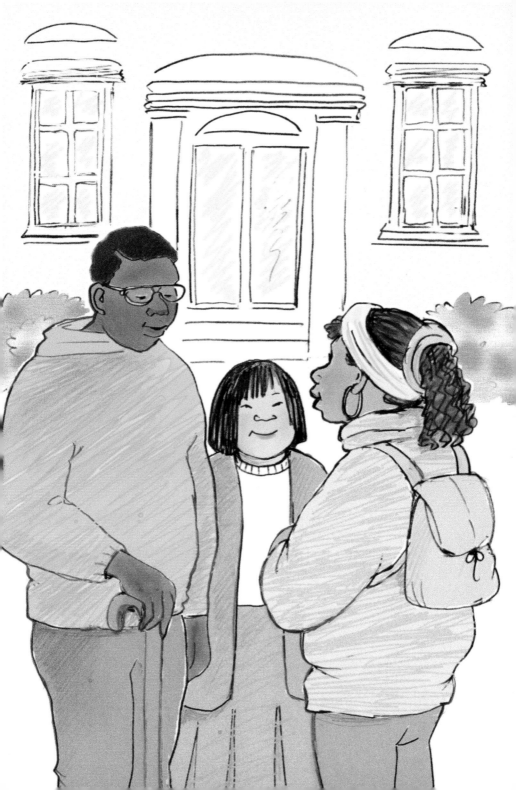

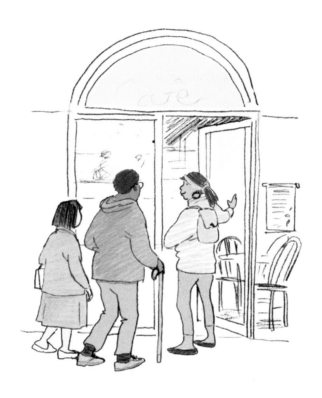

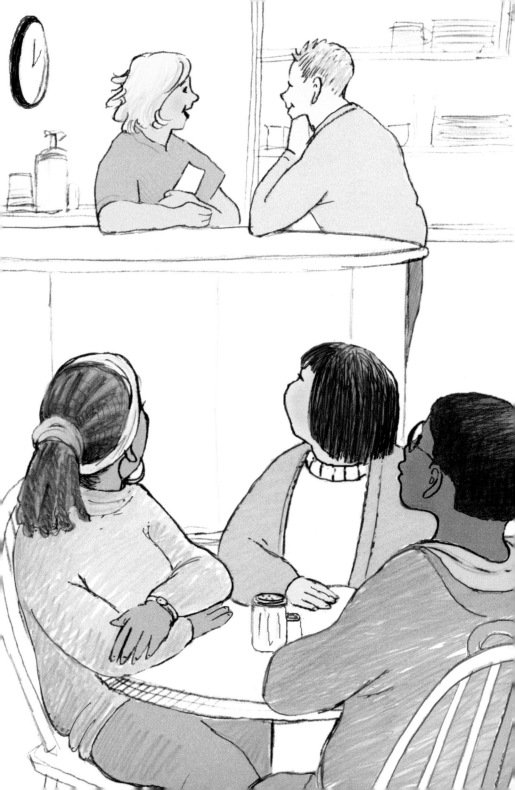

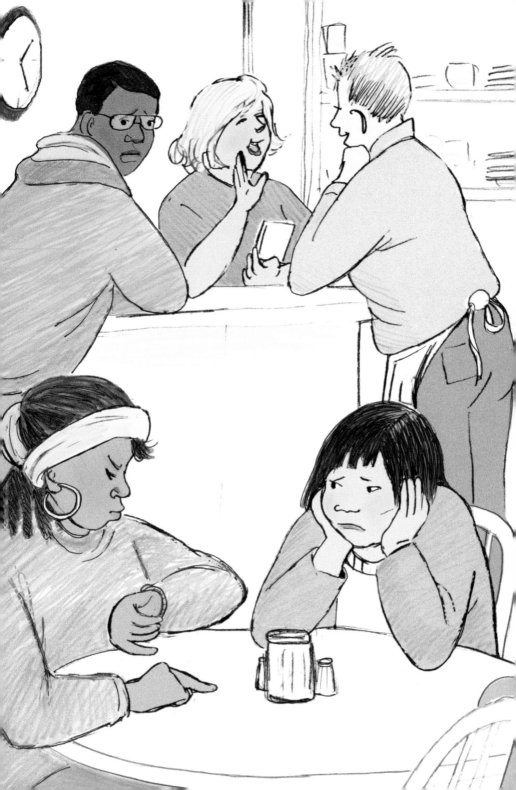

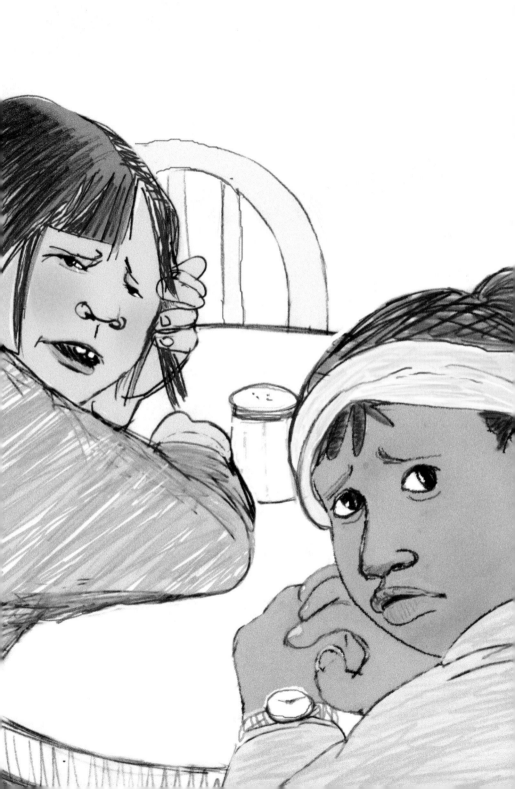

5

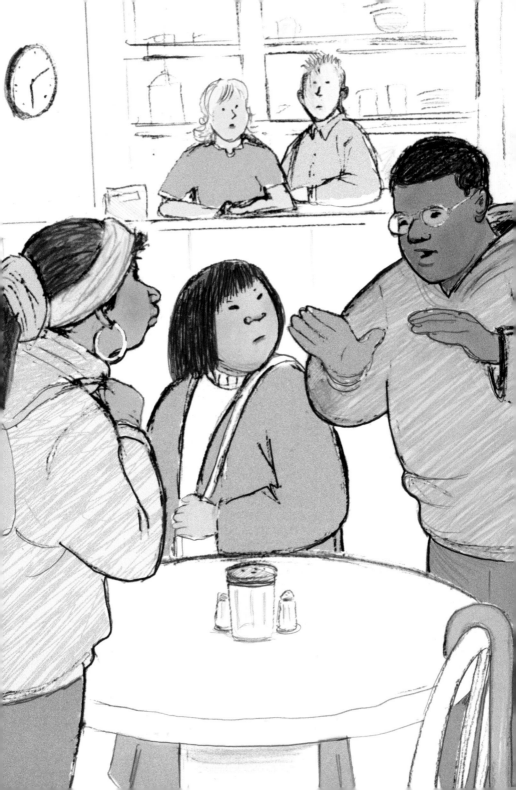

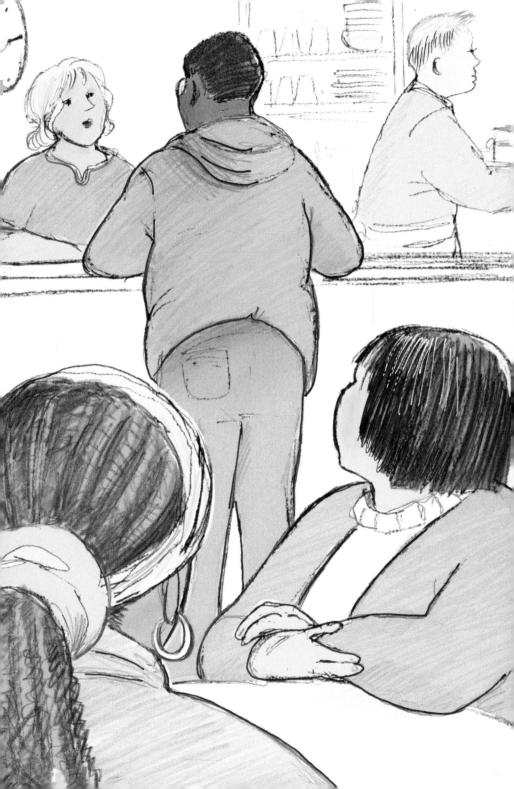

7

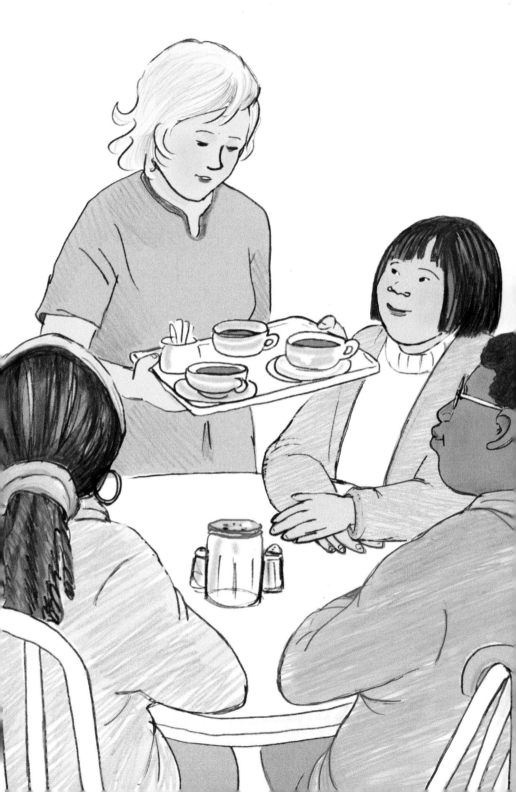

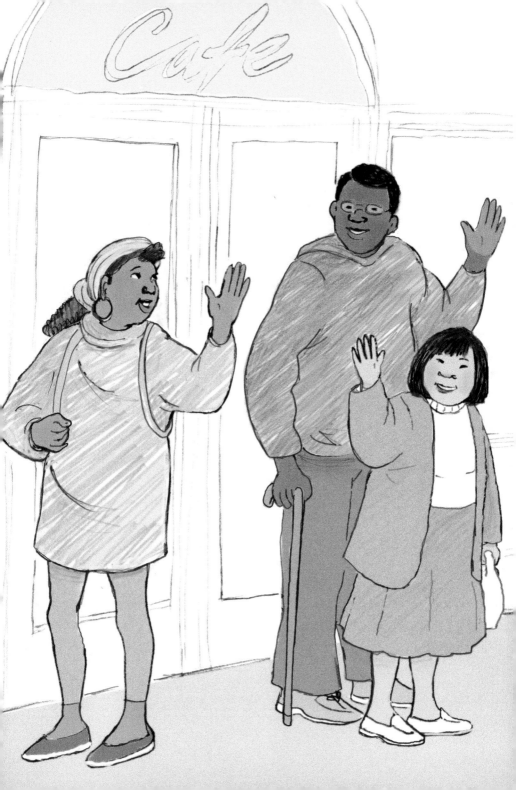

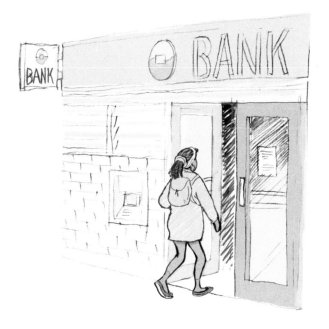

9

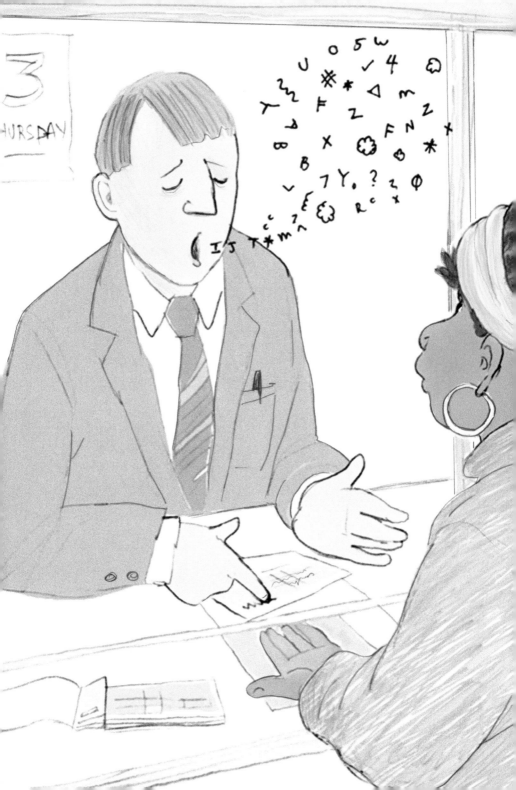

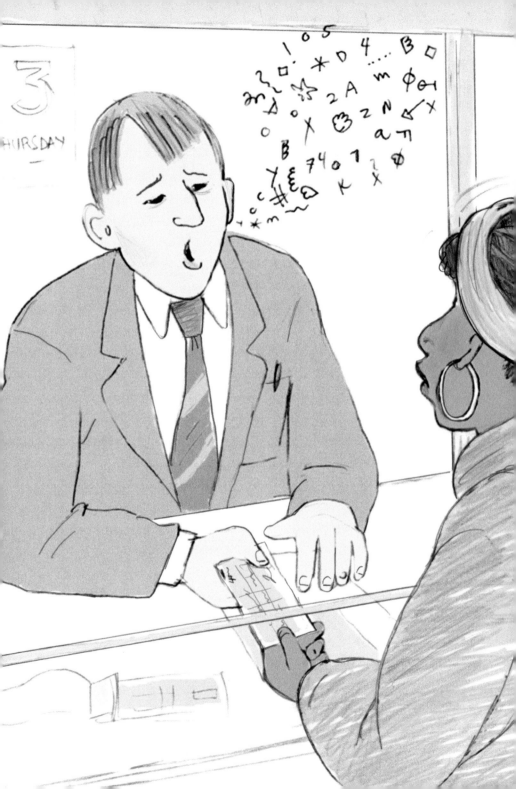

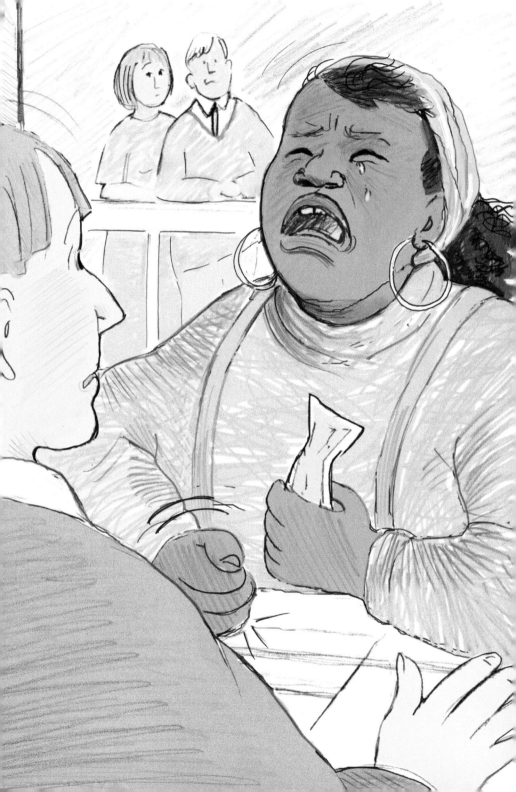

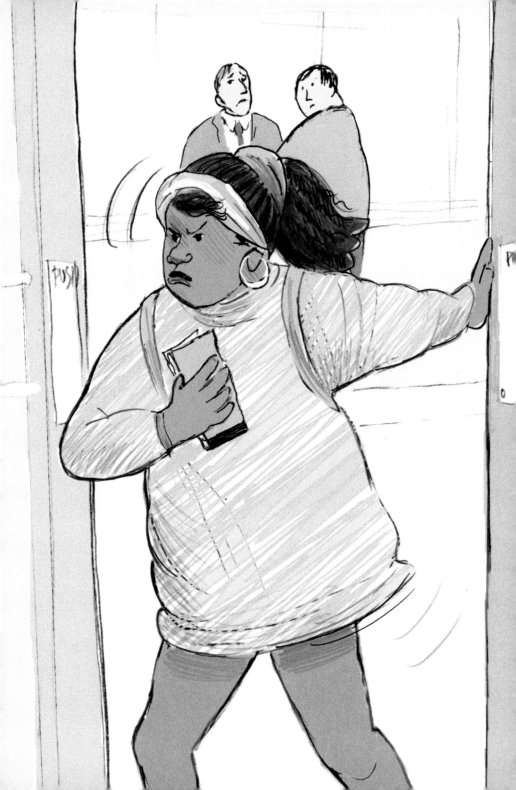

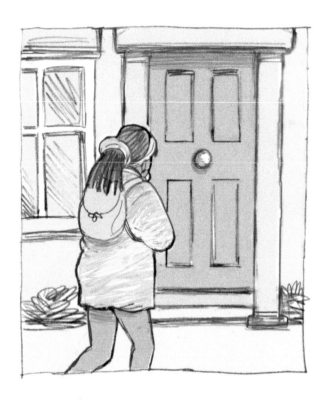

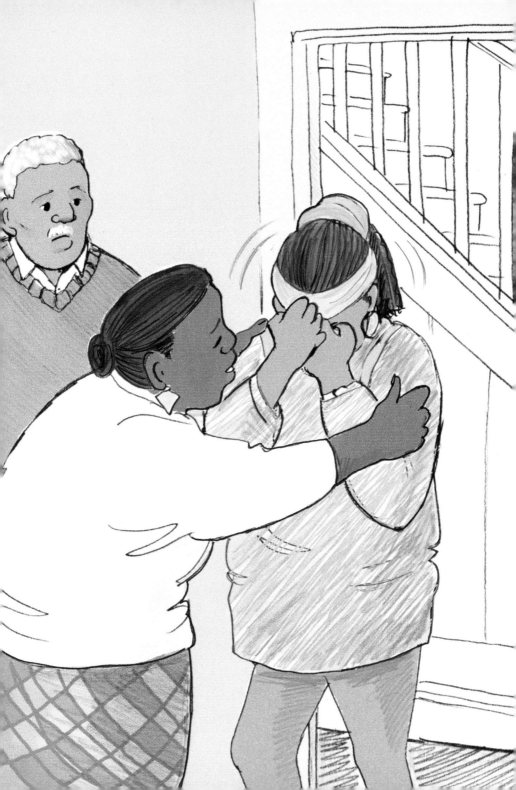

14

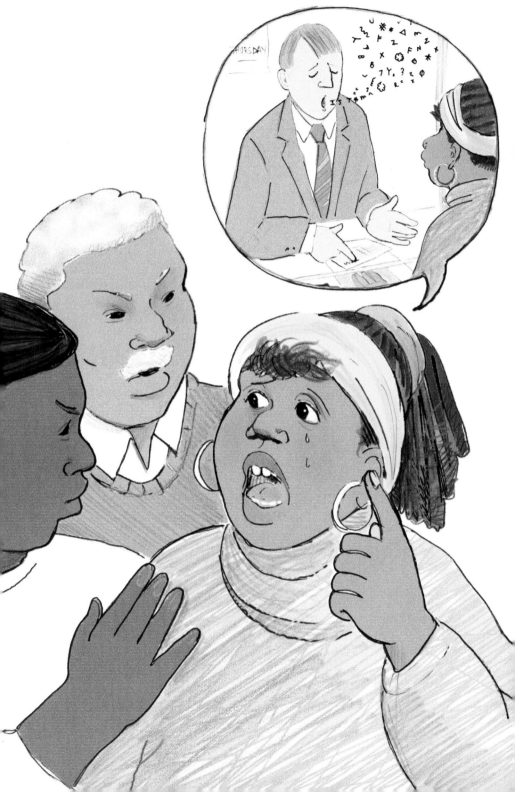

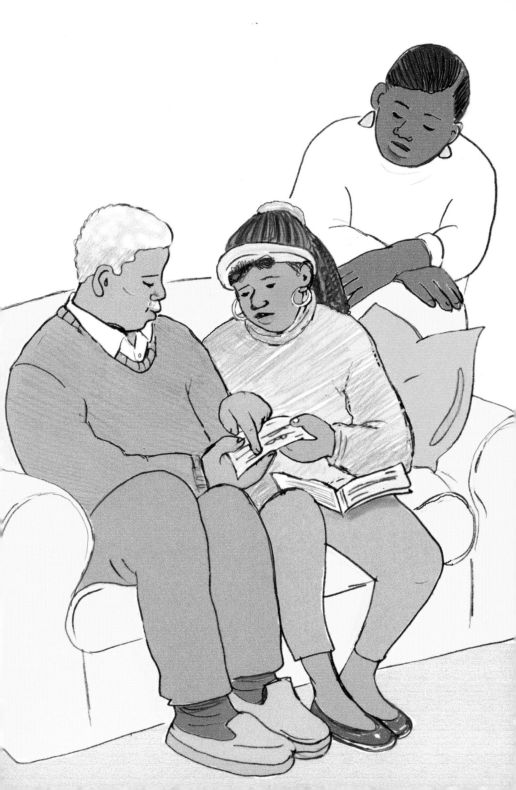

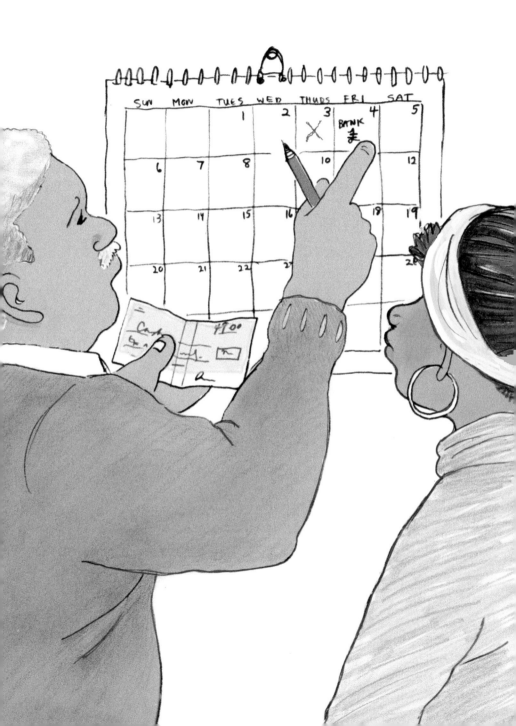

17

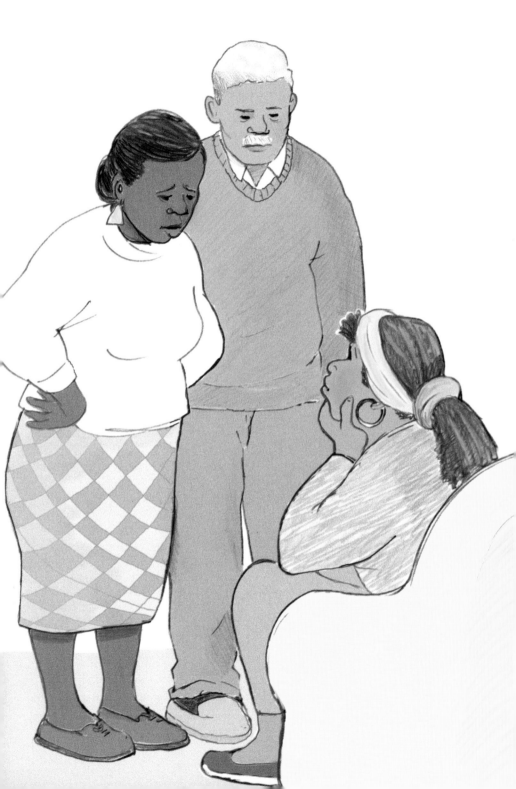

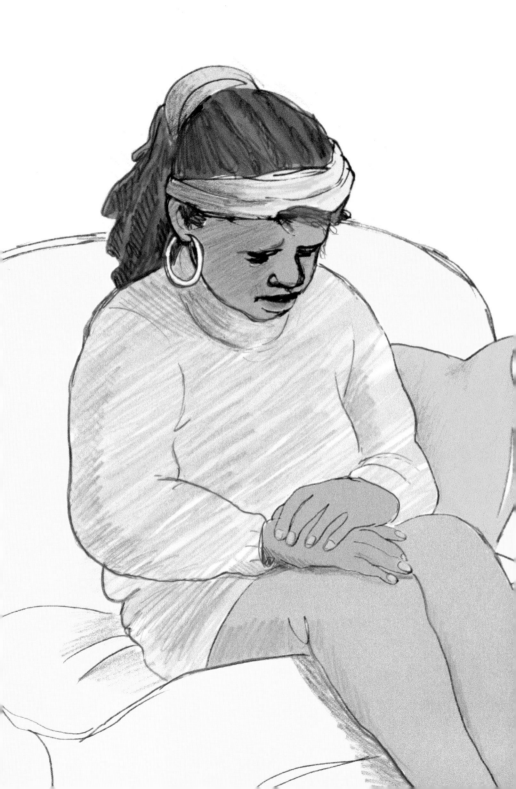

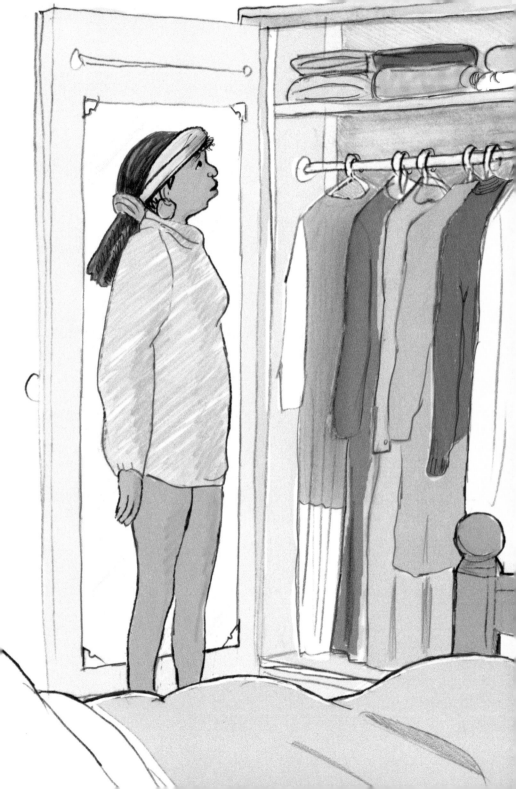

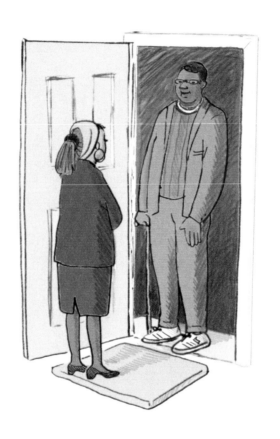

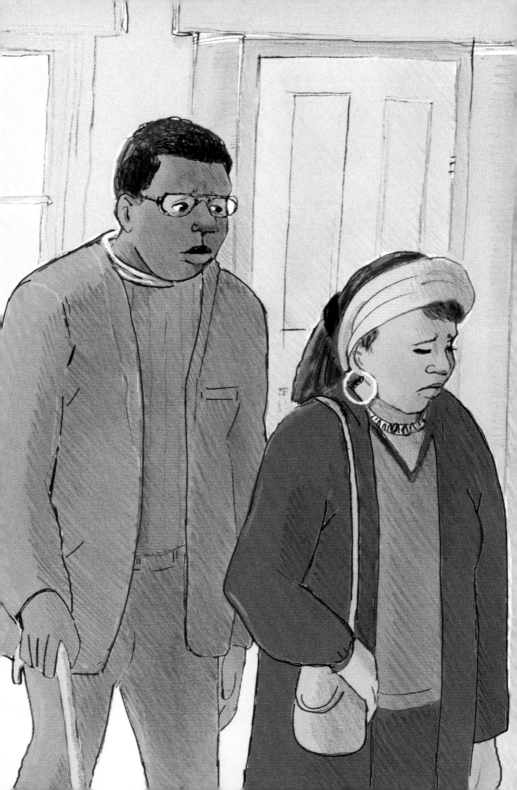

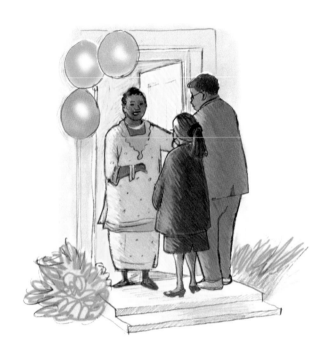

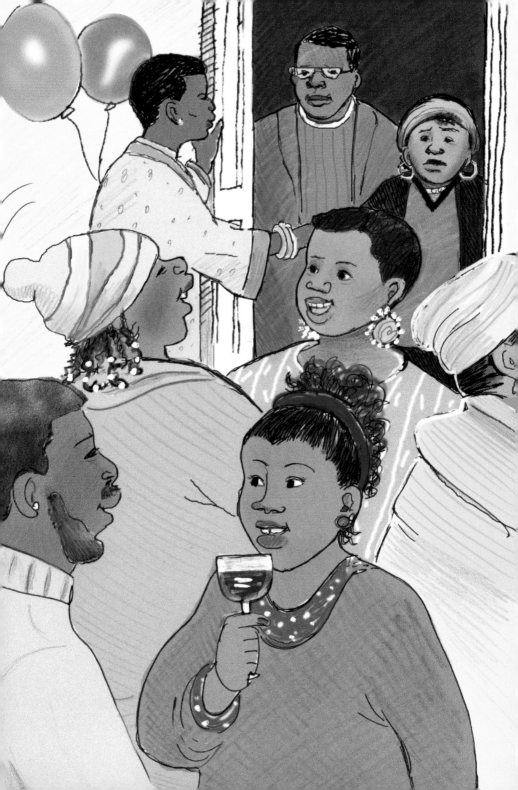

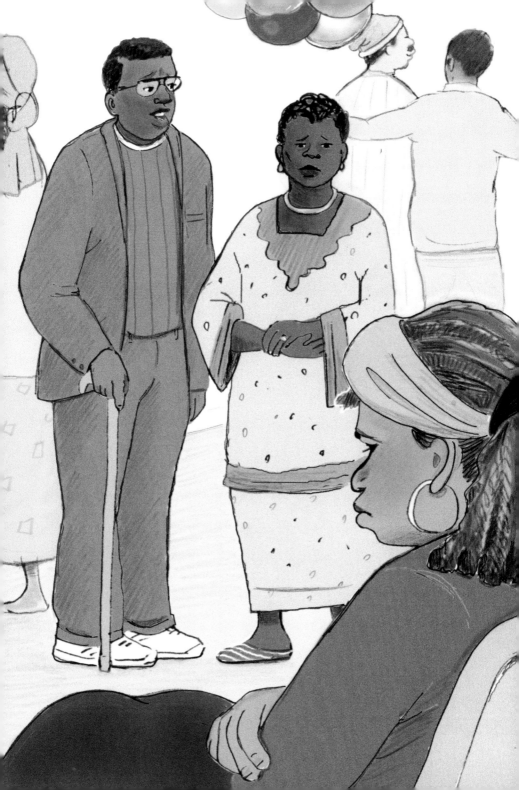

23

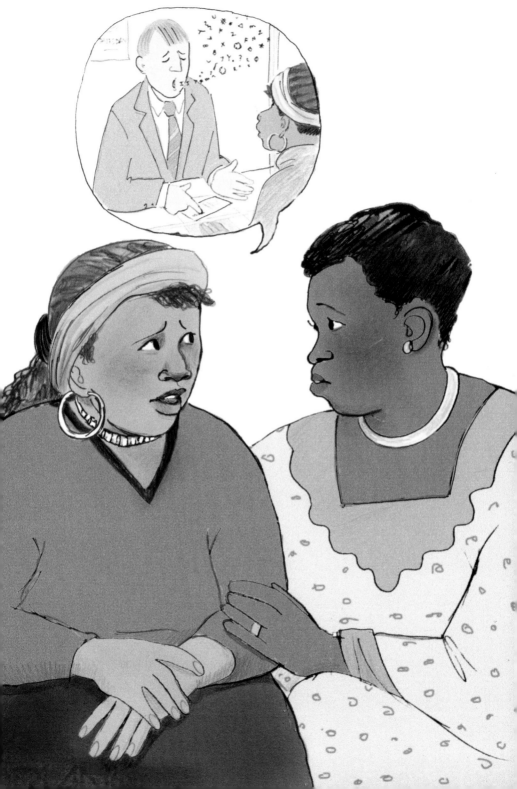

24

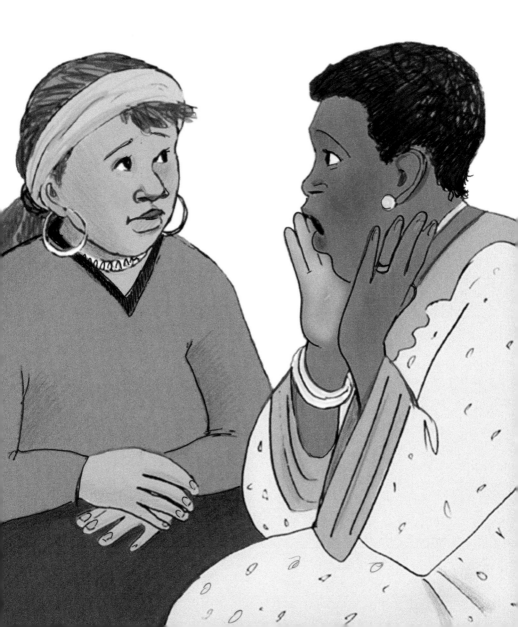

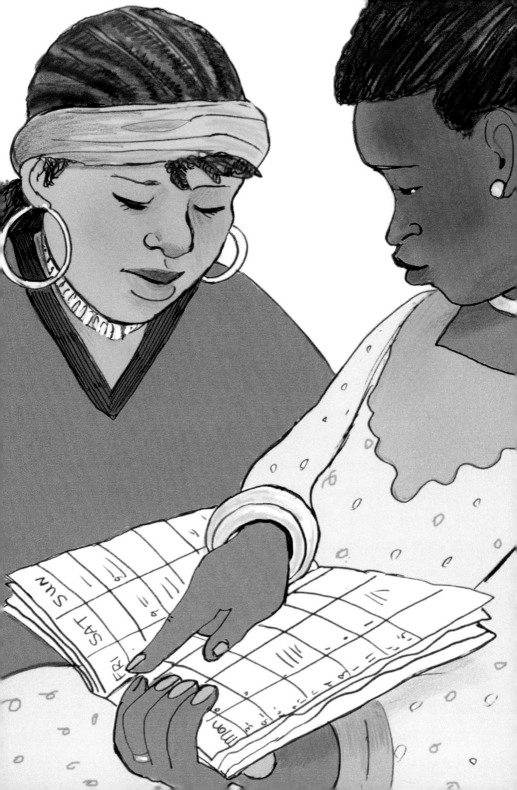

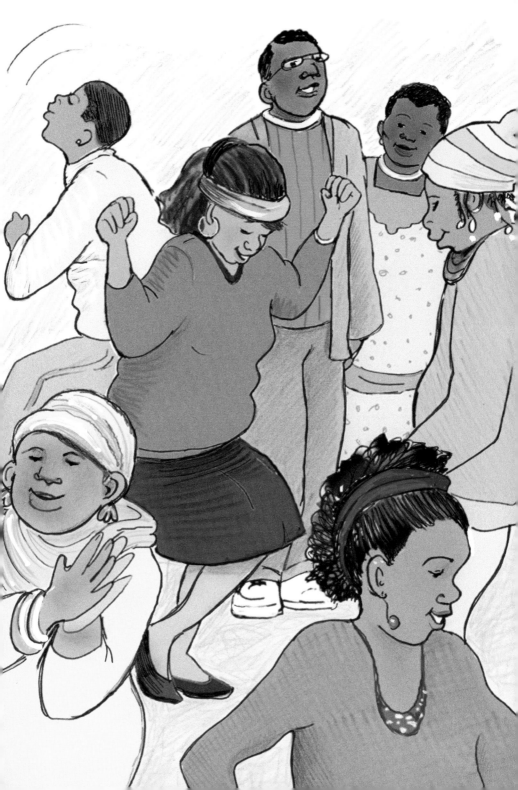

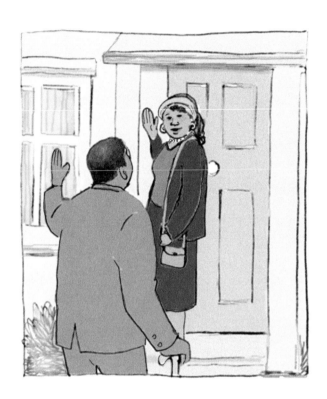

27

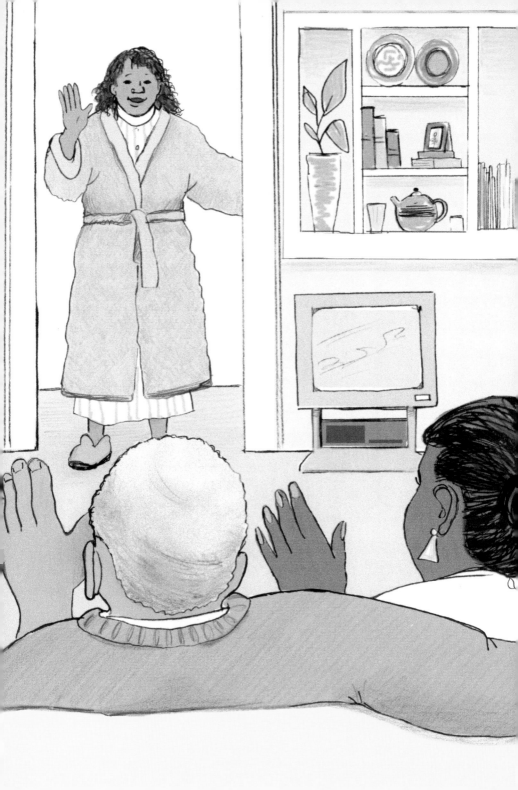

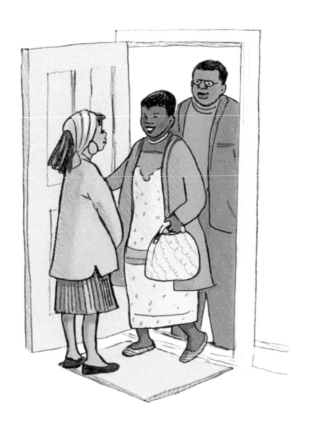

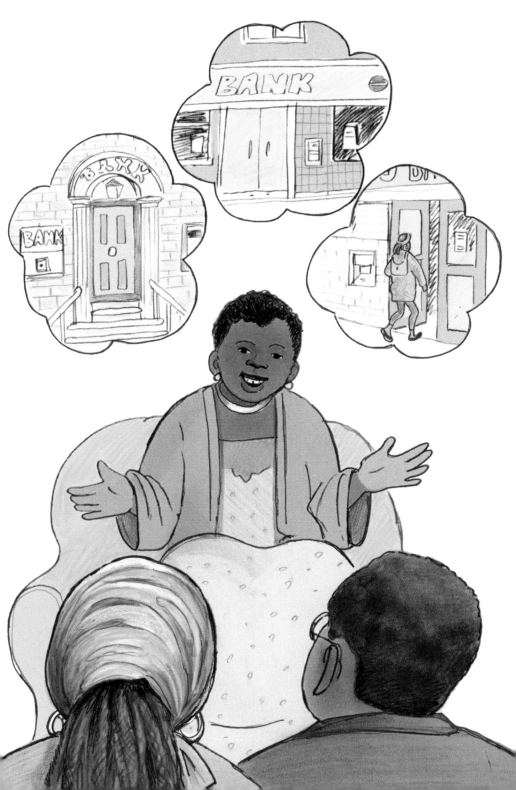

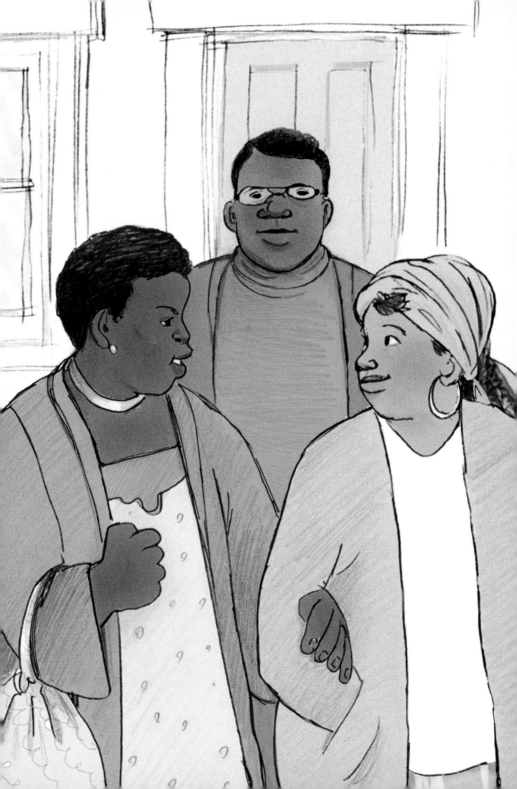

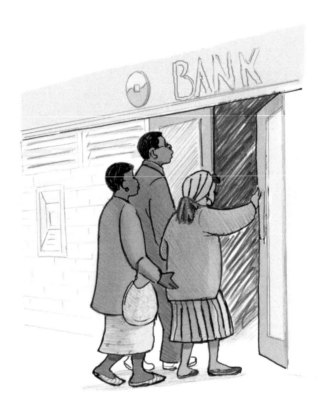

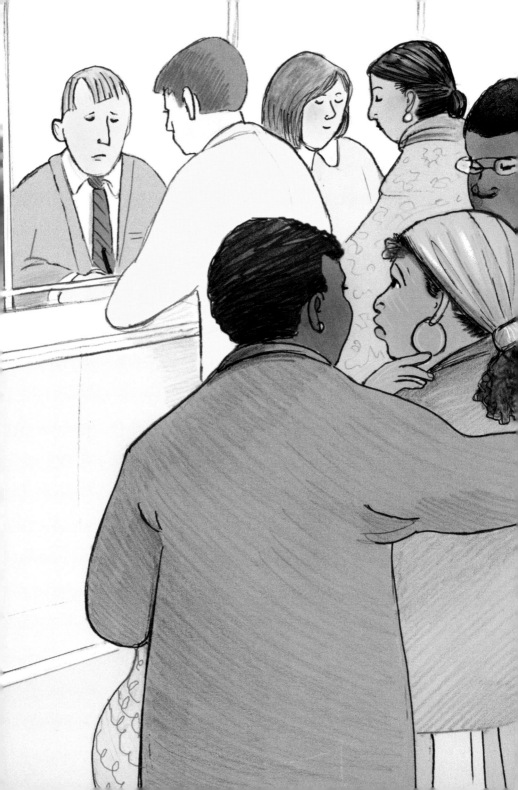

31

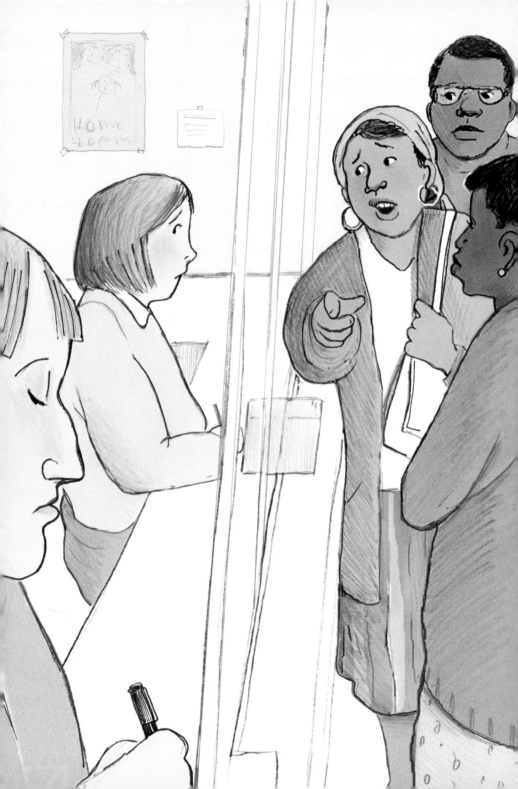

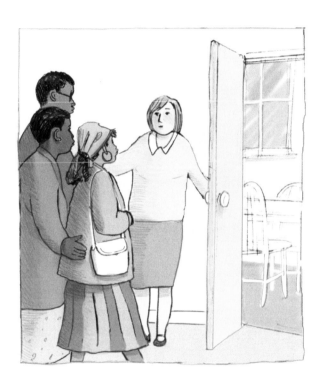

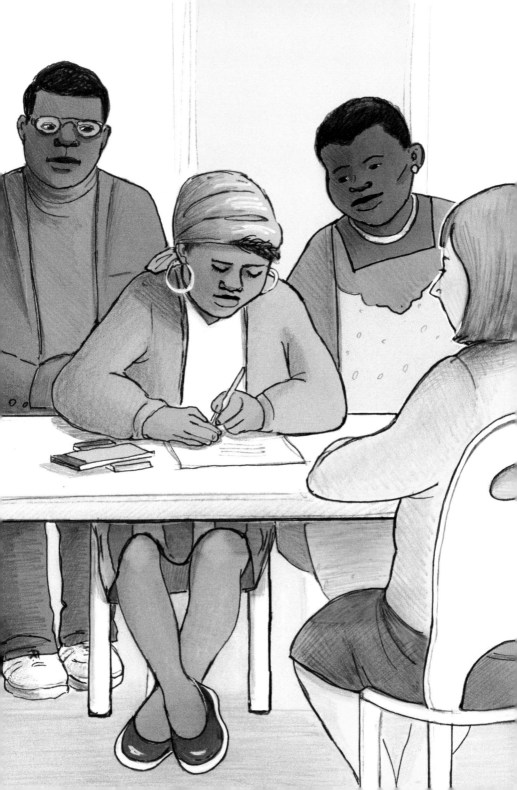

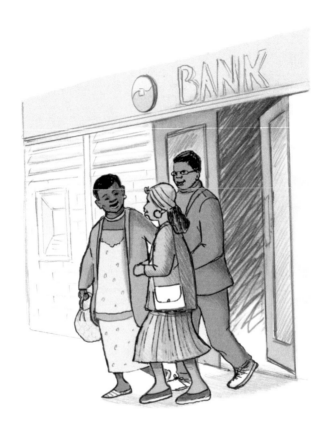

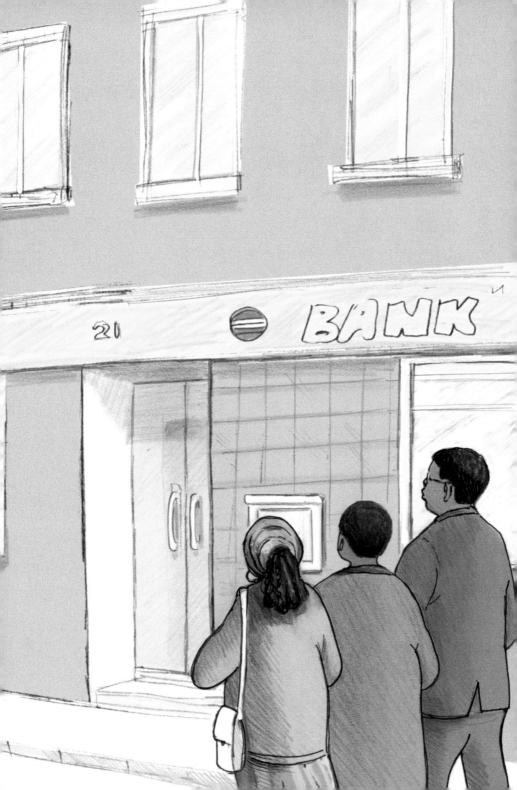

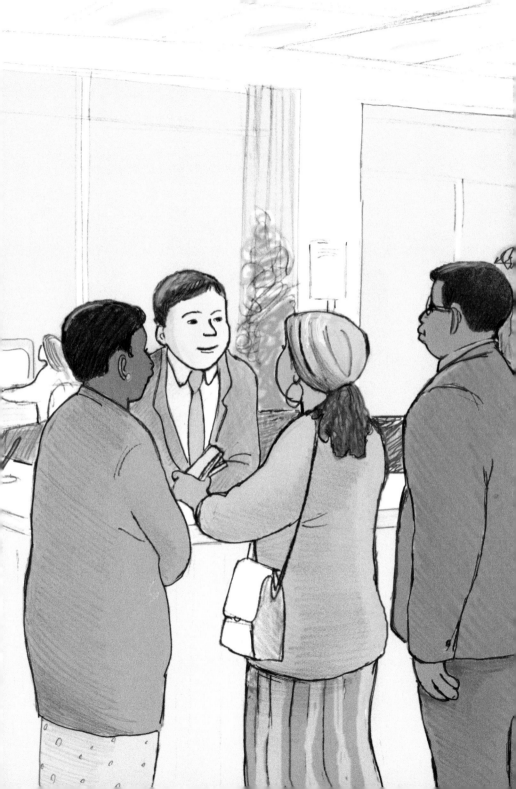

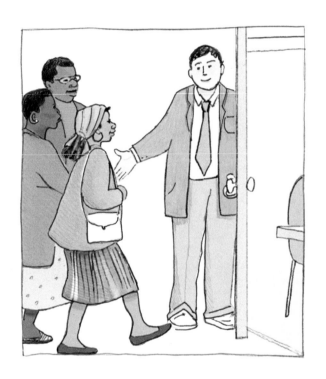

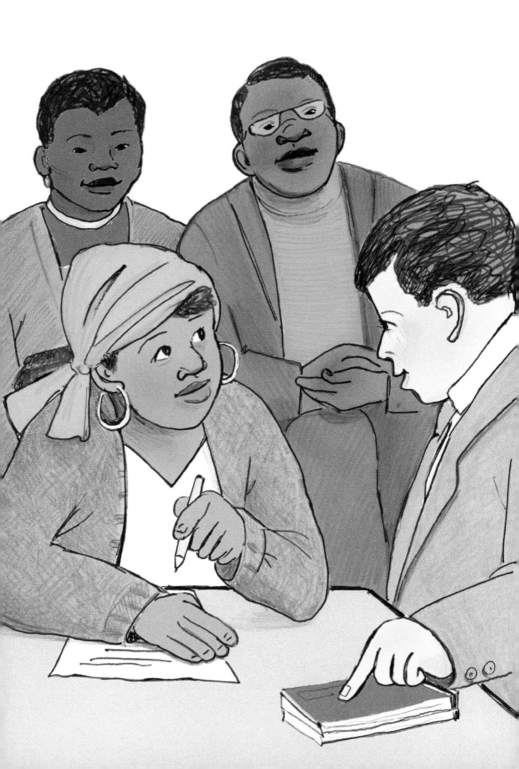

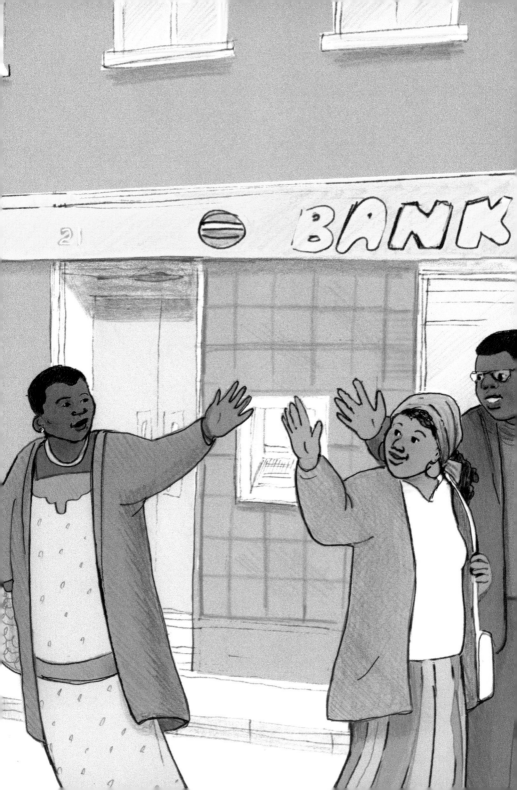

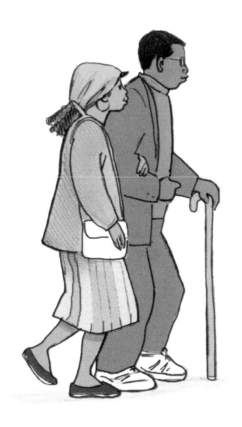

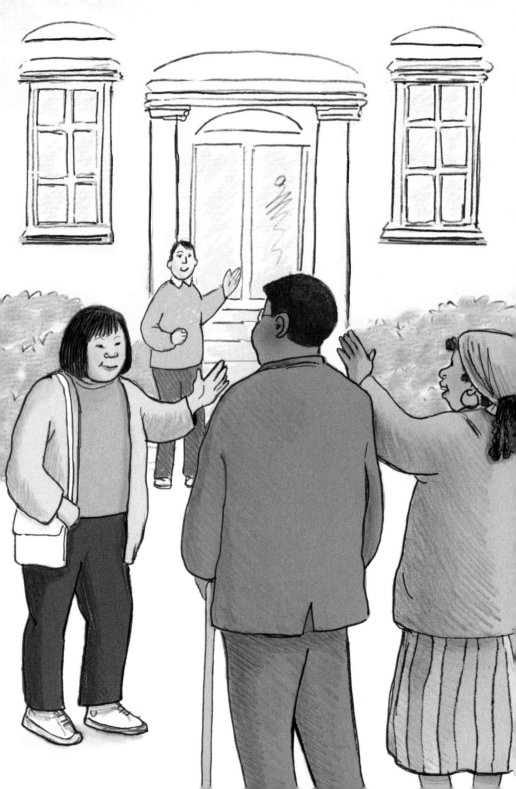

The following words are provided for people who want a ready-made story rather than to tell their own.

1. Natalie, Ben and Susan meet up.

2. They go to a café together. The friends wait for the waitress.

3. They wait for a long time. Ben goes to the counter. The waitress ignores him.

4. They are really fed up. It's bad service.

5. Natalie and Susan say 'Let's go. We don't want to wait.' Ben says 'No. I'll try again.'

6. Ben goes to the counter again. He asks for service.

7. The waitress comes over with the drinks.

8. It's time to go. They say goodbye.

9. Natalie goes to the bank. The bank person speaks jargon. Natalie wants some money. He won't give her any money.

10. He gives her back the cheque. He says 'It's not right.'

11. Oh, he upset her, look! She's crying.

12. Natalie comes out of the bank. She's cross.

13. Natalie goes home. She's with her parents, crying.

14. Natalie tries to tell them what happened. The bank man was hard to understand.

15. Dad tells her 'Look at today's date.' They look at the date on the cheque.

16. Dad says 'Can you remember? You go on a Friday, not Thursday.' They look at the calendar.

17. They're still talking about it.

18. It goes over and over in her head. I don't want to go to that bank again!

19. Natalie is getting ready to go out. She can't decide what to wear.

20. Ben comes to her house. He wonders what's wrong.

21. Natalie and Ben go to a party.

22. Natalie is not joining in. Her friends are worried.

23. Natalie tells Maria about her worries. 'He spoke to me bad. He was speaking in jargon. I went on the wrong day, he was horrible.'

24. Maria says 'That's awful!'

25. Maria is looking in her diary. She and Natalie are going to meet again.

26. Natalie is dancing now.

27. Natalie says goodbye to Ben. She's had a good time. She says goodnight to her parents.

28. Maria arrives with Ben. She tells Ben and Natalie that there are different banks. 'You have a choice.'

29. They're going to the bank. Maria says 'Don't worry, Natalie. We're going to sort everything out!'

30. They arrive at the bank. Natalie's looking scared because of what's happened before.

31. She tells a different bank person 'It's him that was horrible to me.'

32. The bank person listens to Natalie and Maria. She takes them into a side room. She helps Natalie to close her account.

33. They leave the bank. Natalie's happy. They all go on to a different bank.

34. They tell Peter, the new bank person, that Natalie wants to open an account. He asks questions and smiles.

35. Peter shows them round the bank. He is friendly and helpful. He tells Natalie to 'Sign here.' She has a new account!

36. They say 'Hooray, we've done it!' Natalie thanks Maria for coming. They say goodbye.

37. Natalie and Ben feel good about what has happened. They can't wait to tell their friends!

Feeling different

Feeling different can be frightening, upsetting and infuriating. This book is about being made to feel different when asking for a service. If people with intellectual disabilities from ethnic minority groups are discriminated against when they try to use services, they have the right to challenge the service provider. This book will help people to understand their rights. It is wrong to discriminate against anybody for any reason.

People with intellectual disabilities may not know that they should have equal rights to services and the right to be treated with respect. Some people in society do not treat others with respect, especially if they see them as being different from themselves. It's important for people to speak up so that they can change how services are planned and delivered to meet their needs. People may be discriminated against because they have intellectual disabilities. Discrimination can also happen when a service user is from a different ethnic group to the person providing the service. The combination of having an intellectual disability and being from an ethnic minority group feels like a 'double whammy'. It can make it even more difficult to get a good service.

Remember that sometimes discrimination can happen because of a misunderstanding. It is important that people don't jump to the conclusion that they are being discriminated against. Remember that some service providers are not culturally competent.

This book shows two situations where the characters in the story have to overcome difficulties in getting a good service. The first part is set in a café where Ben, Natalie and Susan are treated unacceptably. Through Ben's assertiveness and refusal to give up, they are able to get the service they want.

It shows people can speak up for themselves and do not just have to tolerate discriminatory behaviour. This part of the book can be used to help people understand that not only do they have a voice and the right to be heard, but they also have a choice about how they want to be treated.

The second part of the book shows how Natalie involves someone she knows from her own community in solving a somewhat more complex problem with her bank. The advocate makes it clear to Natalie that she does not have to accept an unsatisfactory service. She is then supported in exercising her choice to go to another bank. This part of the book shows that if someone with intellectual disabilities is not satisfied with a service, but finds it too difficult to deal with on their own, they can involve someone else they trust to represent their views.

There are countless other situations to which the principles illustrated here can be applied, for example in using health services. Just some examples of how problems can be solved are shown here. Other ways include involving friends or relatives, paid carers, citizen advocates (see next page), professionals such as social workers – whoever is most appropriate at the time.

Glossary

Advocacy

Advocacy enables people to express their wishes and aspirations and make real choices. An advocate is someone who gives support to the person who needs their situation to be heard. This role can apply in helping someone access organisations and services such as education, healthcare, social welfare or housing.

Self-advocacy

Self-advocacy means getting your views across by speaking up for yourself and representing your own interests. With the right support, many people with intellectual disabilities can learn to advocate for themselves.

Citizen advocates

Citizen advocates are volunteers who create a relationship with a person with intellectual disabilities, seeking to understand and represent their views. They can make a vital contribution in enabling the voices of people with more complex disabilities to be heard.

Speaking up groups

'Speaking up groups' are good starting points for people who want to learn the skills of speaking up. This is especially important for people who have been denied the right to be involved in the decisions made about their own lives. Groups can be contacted through organisations such as People First in the UK and Values into Action (see the following pages).

Organisations to contact for help in the UK

Where to contact for help and advice

Values into Action (VIA)

Oxford House
Derbyshire Street
London
E2 6HG

Tel: 020 7729 5436
Fax: 020 7729 7797

Email: general@viauk.org
Website: www.viauk.org

Actively campaigns across the UK to promote the rights of people with learning difficulties to equal citizenship. Provides advice, support and grants to help people with learning disabilities to develop self-advocacy groups.

British Institute of Learning Disabilities (BILD)

Campion House
Green Street
Kidderminster
Worcestershire DY10 1JL

Tel: 01562 723 010
Fax: 01562 723 029

Website: www.bild.org.uk
Email: enquiries@bild.org.uk

Works to improve the quality of life for people with learning disabilities through research, education, information and publications. Provides support to citizen advocates working with people with learning disabilities.

Citizen Advocacy Information and Training

162 Lee Valley Technopark
Ashley Road
London N17 9LN

Tel: 020 8880 4545
Fax: 020 8880 4113
(mark f.a.o. CAIT)

Email: cait@teleregion.co.uk

National information resource for citizen advocacy. Citizen advocacy is freely given friendship to vulnerable people.

Equality and Human Rights Commission

Website: www.equalityhumanrights.com

One of the key aims of the Comission is to end discrimination and harassment of people because of their disability. The Disability Discrimination Act 2005 requires services to make 'reasonable adjustments' to support disabled people to make use of their services. If you think you are being discriminated against, you can contact the Commission officess by telephone or by email at the following:

England
Helpline: 0845 604 6610
Email: englandhelpline@equalityhumanrights.com

Wales
Helpline: 0845 604 8810
Email: waleshelpline@equalityhumanrights.com

Scotland
Helpline: 0845 604 5510
Email: scotlandhelpline@equalityhumanrights.com

People First

Unit 3.46 Canterbury Court   Tel: 020 7820 6655
Kennington Park Business Centre Fax: 020 7820 6621
1–3 Brixton Road
London SW9 6DE

Website: www.peoplefirstld.com
Email: general@peoplefirstltd.com

Race Equality Foundation

Unit 35 Kings Exchange   Tel: 0207 619 6220
Tileyard Road   Fax: 0207 619 6230
London N7 9AH

Website: www.raceequalityfoundation.org.uk

Provides race equality consultancy research, development and training in social care.

Circles Network

Potford's Dam Farm
Coventry Road
Cawston
Rugby
Warwickshire CV23 9JP

Tel: 01788 816 671
Fax: 01788 816 672

Website: www.circlesnetwork.org.uk
Email: information@circlesnetwork.org.uk

Provides support and counselling to people with learning disabilities through circles of support.

Written materials

It's Your Choice
By Stephanie Beamer and Mark Brookes (2001). Find out about your right to make your own choices; find out how to get support to make decisions. Workbook and audiotape available from Values into Action at £5.00.

Communicating Choices
Two manuals of signs from the Signalong vocabulary developed to support self-advocacy. *It's My Life* contains 871 signs dealing with, for example, body awareness, social development and coping with abuse and crime. *Independent Living* has 531 signs relating to taking responsibility for the home and taking part in society, for example, shopping, transport and outings, and social notices. Price £30 per copy.

Books Beyond Words

A range of other titles are available in this series.

Three books cover access to criminal justice as a victim (witness) or as a defendant: *Supporting Victims*, *You're Under Arrest* and *You're On Trial*.

Mugged tells what happens to a young man after he is attacked in the street. It includes suggestions for role-playing different responses to unwelcome approaches from strangers. The difficult subject of sexual abuse is covered in *Jenny Speaks Out* and *I Can Get Through It*. Counselling and psychotherapy after sexual abuse are explained in the second title.

Using health services is explained in *Going to the Doctor*, *Going to Out-Patients* and *Going into Hospital*. *Looking After My Breasts* and *Keeping Healthy 'Down Below'* are about breast and cervical screening. *Getting On With Epilepsy* shows how to enjoy an active and independent life with epilepsy. *Getting On With Cancer* deals honestly with the unpleasant side of treatment, but ends on a positive note. *Looking After My Balls* shows young men with intellectual disabilities how to check their testicles to look for anything that may be wrong, and to seek help from their GP if they are worried. *Looking After My Heart* shows how we can prevent heart disease if we make simple and practical changes to our lifestyle.

Am I Going to Die? deals honestly and movingly with the physical and emotional aspects of dying. In *When Somebody Dies*, a man and a woman are helped to feel less sad and to cope with life better after someone they love dies. *When Dad Died* and *When Mum Died* take and honest and straightforward approach to death and grief in the family.

Enjoying Sport and Exercise helps people to choose what activity they would like to do and how to find out what is available to them locally. *Food...Fun, Healthy and Safe* shows how choosing, cooking and eating food can be fun as well as healthy and safe.

Michelle Finds a Voice shows how Michelle and her carers are helped to overcome her difficulties in communication. Various solutions are explored, including the use of signing, symbols and charts.

Speaking Up for Myself shows how people with intellectual disabilities from ethnic minority groups have the right to challenge discrimination.

Falling in Love traces the ups and downs of a romantic relationship.

Two books about personal care are *George Gets Smart* and *Susan's Growing Up*. The latter tells the story of a young girl's first menstruation.

The following Books Beyond Words are now out of print: *Bob Tells All*, *Feeling Blue*, *Hug Me Touch Me*, but their full content can be viewed on www.rcpsych.ac.uk/bbw

The books cost £10 each. To order copies or a leaflet giving more information about these books, please contact: Book Sales, Royal College of Psychiatrists, 17 Belgrave Square, London SW1X 8PG. Credit card orders can be taken by telephone (+44 (0)20 7235 2351, ext. 146). You can also order the books online at http://www.rcpsych.ac.uk/bbw